KETOGENIC DIET

COOKBOOK

99+ Ultimate Recipes To Making Low Carb, High Fat, Weight Loss Paleo Meals For A Healthy Body

(Weight Watchers Book 3)

BY

Virginia A. Caldwell

E-book Edition

First published in 2016

ISBN-13: 978-1537249216

ISBN-10: 1537249215

For more of my awesome cookbooks and recipes please visit my author central page:

amazon.com/author/virginiacaldwell

Table of Contents

Introduction

I want to say a big thank you to everyone who took interest in downloading the book **KETOGENIC DIET COOKBOOK: 99+ Ultimate Recipes To Making Low Carb, High Fat, Weight Loss Paleo Meals For A Healthy Body**.

A ketogenic diet is basically a diet consisting of naturally 75% fat, 20% protein and 5% carbohydrates. But it can essentially differ to about 80% fat, 10% carbohydrates and 10% proteins — or in the ratio 70% fat, 20% protein and 10% carbs. The carbs are quite negligible so your body burns fat rather than sugar to derive energy. This means there is a tiny amount of sugar in your system hindering the body from making use of the fat in favor of burning sugar.

For individuals who need to understand what this book is about: the most important benefit of following a ketogenic diet is that it increases the body's ability to utilize fats for fuel.

It is also a great diet for individuals that suffer from food addiction or binge eating as you may sometimes forget to eat as the ketone bodies diminishes hunger pangs.

For individuals suffering from any blood pressure complications, embarking on this diet is a very good way to:

- Lower blood pressure
- Aid weight loss
- Aid the treatment of Alzheimer's disease
- It is also favorable for individuals suffering with type 2 diabetes who are not on insulin

Note: it would be great if you underwent a full blood lipid panel test prior to going on this plan. This is so that you can compare the "before" and "after" results of your blood work.

If you enjoy reading this book please endeavor to leave a positive review at the customer review section below.

Rösti Hash Browns

Ingredients

- 2 celery roots

- Coconut oil, lard or ghee

- Pepper and salt to taste

- Any preferred topping

Preparation

1. Use a vegetable peeler or paring knife to peel the celery root.

2. Cut the celery into bits then use a food processor or hand grater to grate it.

3. Put pepper and salt to taste.

4. Over average-high heat, heat the oil in a frying pan.

5. You may decide fill your pan and prepare one big Rösti which can be chopped into wedges to ease serving), or you can prepare single smaller hash brown patties.

6. Cook each side for about 15-25 minutes before turning it over to the other side. Do not turn to the other side until the first side is thoroughly browned at the bottom. If you had filled your pan to make a big Rösti, turning it to the other side is easier. You can do that by flipping it onto a plate and then returning it back to the pan.

7. Allow to cook additional 12- 17 minutes till it has browned as before.

8. Serve with tomato salsa, roasted vegetables, bacon or scrambled or fried eggs.

Baked Sugar Detox Cookies

Ingredients

- Sugar-free almond butter, 1cup

- Coconut oil, 4 teaspoons

- 4 eggs

- Vanilla extract, 1 teaspoon

- Cinnamon, 2 teaspoons

- Coconut flour, 2 tablespoons

- Pecans (diced), ½ cup

- Unsweetened shredded coconut, 2 cups

Preparation

1. Firstly heat the oven to 350F

2. Use silicone mat or parchment paper to line a baking sheet

3. If necessary, melt the coconut oil

4. Stir vanilla, eggs, coconut oil and almond butter together inside a mixing bowl. Stir thoroughly to ensure that the ingredients combine well. This part is a bit difficult.

5. Gently add the coconut flour and cinnamon and stir in till it is properly blended, afterwards put in the pecans and shredded coconut.

6. Transfer to baking sheet in little clumps. It will be able to reach 16-20 depending on your scoop size.

7. Use a fork to flatten the clumps to around a quarter inch thickness (you will have to coat the fork with additional coconut flour to prevent it from sticking to the cookies)

8. Bake for 15-20 minutes.

9. Make sure you don't over-bake in order to prevent the clumps from drying out.

Non-Fat Cinnamon Bun Bars

Ingredients

- Creamed coconut sliced into chunks, 1 cup

- Cinnamon, ½ teaspoon

First Icing:

- Un-dissolved coconut oil (extra virgin), 2 tablespoons

- Almond butter, 2 tablespoons

- Second Icing:

- Almond butter or coconut oil, 2 tablespoons

- Cinnamon, 1 tablespoon

Preparation

1. Use the suitable liner to line a mini loaf pan or dish.

2. Manually mix cinnamon and coconut cream. Pat into the dish. This should fill 4 mini loaf sections.

3. First Icing: In a separate bowl mix the almond butter and coconut oil together. This should be spread over the creamed coconut. Refrigerate the bars for about 7 or more minutes.

4. Second Icing: In a bowl, mix the icing together. Sprinkle the icing on the bars and either eat or refrigerate again.

5. Cut bar into small chunks with a knife.

Vegan Chicken And Noodle Sauce

Ingredients

- 1 chicken breast, sliced into bits

- 1 medium green onion, diced

- 1½ Tablespoons avocado oil

- 2 cups chicken broth

- ¼ cup cilantro, thinly sliced

- 1 stalk of celery, sliced

- Salt to taste

- 1 zucchini, skinned, chopped

Preparation

1. Pour the avocado oil into the saucepan and stir-fry the chopped chicken until properly done.

2. Pour the chicken broth into the pan and boil.

4. Slice the celery and pour it into the boiling pan.

5. Slice the green onions and stir into the pan.

6. Slice the cilantro and set aside for a while.

7. Prepare the zucchini noodles. Use a potato peeler, food processor or spiralizer to slice it into long strands.

8. Stir in the cilantro and zucchini noodles.

9. Boil for some minutes, season with salt to taste, and serve at once.

Vegan Chicken Paprika

Ingredients

- 2 eggs, whisked

- 1 lb chicken tenders or skinless chicken breast, diced into strips

- 1 teaspoon Paprika

- ¾ cup Almond Meal

- ½ teaspoon powdered Cumin Seed

- ½ teaspoon powdered Coriander Seed

- 1/3 teaspoon Salt

Preparation

1. Preheat the oven to 425 degrees. Use parchment paper to line the inside of a big baking sheet.

2. Mix together the almond meal with the rest spices in a bowl or shallow plate. Pour the whisked egg into a different shallow plate.

3. Pat the chicken dry using a paper towel. Coat the chicken with egg then coat with almond meal mixture, ensure all sides are coated. Arrange on the baking sheet. Do the same for all the other chicken tenders.

4. Bake for about 15 to 20 minutes, flipping it once after half the time of baking is gone, until it is properly cooked.

Paleo Chicken Salad

Ingredients

For marinade

• Vinegar (apple cider), 4 tablespoons

• Olive oil (extra virgin), 4 tablespoons

• Chopped dried thyme, 2 teaspoons

• Garlic (granulated), 2 teaspoons

• Salt to taste, 2 teaspoons

• Pepper, 2 teaspoons

For Salad

• Average-sized avocados (shredded and minced), 4

• Mayo (Primal Kitchen brand), 4 tablespoons

• Chicken breast (boneless and without skin), 3 pounds

• Shredded celery, 6 stalks

• Olives (diced), kalamata or black, ½ cup

• Cilantro or parsley (diced), 4 tablespoons

• 2 Tomatoes, minced

• Pepper and salt to taste

• Romaine leaves

Preparation

FOR MARINADE

1. Put all the ingredients in a bowl, followed by the chicken breasts and mix. Refrigerate for a minimum of 20 minutes, but it can take about 24 hours to marinade in an air tight container.

FOR SALAD

1. In a large bowl, squash minced avocado and mix in mayo.

2. After about 20 minutes of the chicken breasts being in the marinade, grill the chicken or bake it till it is fully cooked. Allow it to cool and proceed to chop.

3. Pour the herbs, olives, celery, tomato (based on choice), chicken, pepper and salt to the mayo/avocado mixture. To combine, mix them.

Fat Bomb Easter Egg Cookies

Ingredients

- 5-10 drops alcohol-free stevia

- 3 cups Bob's Red Mill Almond Flour

- ½ cup sugar-free dark chocolate chips

- 1 cup coconut oil, dissolved

- ½ teaspoon gray sea salt

- 1 ½ teaspoon alcohol-free vanilla extract

Coating

- Easter-themed natural food coloring

- 1 cup coconut butter, dissolved

Preparation

1. Line the inside of a baking sheet with silicon baking mat or parchment paper.

2. Pour in the coconut oil, almond flour, stevia, vanilla, and salt into the S-bladed food processor. Puree for roughly 20 seconds or until very smooth.

3. Stir in the chocolate chips. Spoon about 2 tablespoons and shape into a ball using your palms. Arrange on the prepared lined baking sheet and compress, turning into a big egg. Repeat the same with the rest of the dough.

4. Place the baking sheet in the freezer and freeze for an hour.

5. Transfer to a cooling rack and set aside.

6. Make the frosting by dissolving the coconut butter, splitting into different dishes, and adding food coloring.

7. Take the keto cookie dough eggs out of the freezer. Plunge only one end of each cookie in the coconut butter and put on the cooling rack. Pour in the rest of the colored coconut butter into a Ziploc bag, tear out a little hole and sprinkle over the top.

8. Place the eggs on the cooling rack in the fridge to solidify for an hour.

9. Store in a sealed container for up to 5 days in the refrigerator. It can be kept frozen for up to a month.

Italian Cheese Meatballs

Ingredients

- White onion, (diced), 2 ounces

- Olive oil, ½ tablespoon

- Cold ricotta cheese (whole milk), ½ cup

- 1 cold big egg

- Granulated garlic, 1 teaspoon

- Italian seasoning, 1 teaspoon

- Sea salt, 1 teaspoon

- Black pepper (freshly ground), ¼ teaspoon

- Chopped romano/parmesan/asiago mix, ½ cup

- Ground beef (80% lean), ½ pound

Preparation

1. Firstly heat the oven to 340F, then use parchment paper to line a cookie sheet to make cleanup less difficult.

2. Fry onions briefly in olive oil till they are semi-transparent, then bring down from the oven and allow it to cool for about 15 minutes.

3. With onions still cooling, dice the chopped Parmesan in a blender till it is crumbled to fine grains. Keep it aside.

4. Mix egg and ricotta cheese in a bowl. Stir till it is smooth.

5. Put the salt, pepper and spices and pepper and stir.

6. Put the diced Parmesan and onions. Stir properly.

7. Add beef and mix until all ingredients are combined.

8. Split the meat mixture into portions of 1 ounce each.

9. Make each portion into the shape of a ball.

10. Put meatballs on a cookie sheet, and bake at 340F till they are thoroughly cooked and brown in color. This should take around half an hour.

Spicy Fillet Frittata

Ingredients

- 6 eggs

- 1 lbs. salmon

- 1 tablespoon cooking oil or butter or ghee

- ¼ of small onion

- 1 tablespoon diced capers

- 1 tablespoon diced dill

- Caper and Dill Mayo

- 1 teaspoon sliced chives

- Salt and pepper to taste

Preparation

1. Preheat the oven to 375 degrees.

2. Pour oil into a big saucepan and heat on medium-high heat

3. Using a scissors, slice the salmon into bits of fillets.

4. Rub pepper and salt on either side of the salmon.

5. When the oil is well heated gently pour the salmon fillets into hot saucepan.

6. Cook for roughly 5 minutes or until the salmon is done two-thirds of the way and doesn't stick to the pan any more. Fry till it's crusty.

7. Toss the salmon and fry for another 3 minutes or until properly done.

8. Turn off the heat.

9. Lightly rub nonstick spray on a baking dish to prevent sticking.

10. In a separate bowl, carefully beat together the eggs, capers, pepper, dill, chives and a dash of salt in another mixing bowl.

11. Shred the salmon fillets into fairly-sized chunks and place in the greased baking dish, you can stack them if they all don't fit at once.

12. Sprinkle the egg mixture over the salmon.

13. Swirl the baking dish slightly to make certain the egg is uniformly spread.

14. Bake for about half an hour at 375 degrees in an oven or until the middle is no longer soggy.

15. Remove from oven and allow it to cool for about 10 minutes before serving.

16. Garnish with Caper and Dill Mayo.

Chicken in Herb Cream Sauce

Ingredients

- Butter, 8 tablespoons, split into different parts

- White onions, 4, shredded

- Garlic cloves, 5 big ones

- Chicken broth, 1 cup

- Dry white wine, 1 cup

- Cream cheese, 12 ounces

- Heavy cream, 1 cup

- Tarragon (dried), 2 teaspoons

- Herbes de Provence, 3 teaspoons

- Chicken seasoning (Weber Canadian brand), 2 teaspoons

- Salt

- 5 Chicken breasts (raw)

Preparation

1. Fry tarragon, garlic and onions, at average heat, in 4 tablespoons of butter till they soften. Bring down from the skillet and keep it aside.

2. Put 2 tablespoons of butter in the skillet used in step 1, and melt at low heat. Pour in the wine. Put the cream cheese and mix till it melts and is thoroughly combined with the butter and wine. Put spices and cream and mix by stirring.

3. Firstly heat the oven to 340F. Grease a baking dish with1 tablespoon of butter. Then pour the chicken broth into the baking dish.

4. Add single layer of chicken to the baking dish.

5. Equally put a spoonful of onion mixture on the chicken.

6. Scoop cream sauce mixture over onions and chicken. Bake at 340F for about 50-60 minutes.

7. Serve alongside a salad.

Confetti Egg And Veggie Salad

Ingredients

- 8 big Eggs, hard boiled, shelled and sliced

- 3 tablespoons Horseradish Mustard

- 1 cup thinly diced Celery

- ½ cup fresh Herbs, thinly sliced

- ½ cup onion, thinly diced

- ¾ cup mayonnaise

- 4 tablespoons sweet pickle relish

- ½ cup thinly sliced Red Pepper

- Sea Salt and Pepper, to taste

Preparation

1. Mix together all the ingredients.

2. Spice with pepper and salt to taste.

3. Serve right away or refrigerate for later consumption.

Portobello Mushroom Caps With Baked Eggs

Ingredients

- Portobello mushroom caps

- Farm-fresh eggs

- A little olive oil

- slices of prosciutto

- Fresh parsley or thyme

- Black pepper

Preparation

1. Wipe the Portobello mushroom caps clean with a moist fabric, cut off the stem and scratch out the gills to make a well deep enough to contain the egg.

2. Coat the outside of the mushroom with a little oil before cooking it to keep it from sticking to the body of the pan. Place the caps on a baking sheet.

3. Put a slice of prosciutto inside the mushroom cap.

4. Crack each egg and pour into a small bowl and then gently drain it into a prosciutto-filled mushroom cap.

5. Drizzle with fresh herbs and black pepper, as desired.

6. Gently put the baking pan inside the 375 degree F pre-heated oven and bake for about 20 to 30 minutes.

Vegan Cauliflower And Pizza Crust

Ingredients

- Olive oil, 2 tablespoons

- 2 big cauliflower (organic), trimmed and diced into bits

- White onion, 3 ounces, diced

- Butter, 4 tablespoons

- Water, ½ cup

- 6 eggs

- Mozzarella cheese (shredded), minced by food processor into tiny pieces.

- Fennel seed, 2 teaspoons

- Italian seasoning, 4 teaspoons

- Grated parmesan, ½ cup

Preparation

1. First heat the oven to 440F. Use olive oil to grease a 17 x 11 cookie sheet.

2. Melt butter in a big skillet that has a cover, and then add cauliflower and onion. Briefly fry the vegetables at low to average heat till cauliflower is nearly done.

3. Pour in the water. Secure the lid and boil till the cauliflower is fully limp. Bring and keep aside to cool.

4. As soon as the cauliflower is cool, put 3 measured cups in a food processor. Blend it till it is smooth. Scratch out the pureed cauliflower and put it in a mixing bowl.

5. Add the cheese, spices, eggs, parmesan cheese and minced mozzarella to the cauliflower. Combine properly.

6. Spread the cauliflower mixture with the help of a spatula on the greased cookie sheet. Spread it in such a way that there is uniform thickness.

7. The crust should then be baked at 440F for around 30 minutes, or till it appears the surface has cooked and has brown edges.

Curried Chicken And Salad

Ingredients

Salad ingredients

• Cooked chicken breast (minced), 3 cups

• Minced celery, 1 cup

• Almonds (sliced), ½ cup

• Green onions (diced), ½ cup

• Carrot (diced), ½ cup

Dressing ingredients

• Thick sour cream, 5 ounces

• Mayonnaise, 5 ounces

• Pepper and salt to taste

• Curry powder, 2 teaspoons

• 3-4 drops of EzSweet liquid splenda or half teaspoon of stevia glycerite

Preparation

1. Mix mayonnaise and sour cream till you get a smooth mixture.

2. Put the seasoning and mix till it's smooth.

Finished Salad:

1. Mix the dressing and salad ingredients and stir properly.

2. Serve.

Buttery Spaghetti with Hazelnuts

Ingredients

- 1 tablespoon room temperature butter

- ¼ cup whole hazelnuts (filberts)

- 1 cup lightly packed boiled spaghetti squash, warmed

- Salt to taste

Preparation

1. Dice the hazelnuts into tiny bits.

2. Dissolve the butter in a medium-sized pan and heat over medium heat.

3. Stir the butter slowly and wait for it to start turning brown. Once it begins to turn brown, turn off the heat under the pan and stir in the diced hazelnuts. Whisk the hazelnuts together with the butter.

4. Drizzle the hazelnut and butter mixture over the squash, spice with salt and serve.

Chicken And Kale Veggie Sauce

Ingredients

- 8 organic carrots, chopped

- 32 ounces organic chicken broth

- 3 big chicken breasts, shredded into strips

- 2 heads celery, chopped

- 2 heads of kale thinly diced, plus the stems

- 2 yellow onion, cubed

- Sea salt and pepper

Preparation

1. Put all the ingredients, aside from the kale inside a big pot and heat over medium heat and boil for around 45 minutes or until the chicken is completely done. When the chicken is properly cooked, it should be easy to shred. You can use tongs or fork to tear the chicken to pieces and into small bits. Next, pour in the kale and stir together.

2. Serve while it is hot.

Herbs And Roasted Radishes

Ingredients

- 2 bunches of radishes, remove stems and slice into quarters

- 2 tablespoon grass-fed tallow

- 2 tablespoon chopped fresh herbs

- 3 tablespoons chopped fresh chives

- Sea salt and powdered pepper, to taste

Preparation

1. Pour the grass-fed tallow into a cast iron pan.

2. Heat the pan over medium heat. Dissolve the tallow, stir in the chopped radishes, powdered pepper and sea salt. Leave it to boil for about 7 minutes.

3. Stir in the fresh chives. Boil for about 2 minutes before pouring in the fresh herbs. Boil for another minute.

4. Serve at once or, leave it to cool fully, then place in a container and store in the refrigerator.

Smoked Radishes And Rosemary

Ingredients

- Radishes (sliced in two), 2 cups

- Sea salt, 1 teaspoon

- Black peppercorns, 6

- Fresh Rosemary (organic), 2 asparagus

- Olive oil, 2 tablespoons

- Stemless radish tops

Preparation

1. Firstly heat oven to about 425F.

2. Cut the stems off of the radish, pick the leaves, and put the leaves aside.

3. Based on their shape and size cut the radishes into either two or four parts. The radishes should be fairly equal in size so as to ensure uniform roasting.

4. Thoroughly grind peppercorns and ½ teaspoon of sea salt using a mortar & pestle.

5. Chop the rosemary.

6. Cover the radishes with rosemary, pepper, 1 tablespoon of olive oil, and salt.

7. Transfer the mixture to a baking sheet (non-stick) and bake at 430F for about 25-32 minutes, or till radishes turn golden and crisp then you bring down from the oven.

8. Heat the rest (1 tablespoon) of the olive oil in a big sauté pan at average heat. Add the remaining ½ teaspoon of salt and the radish top leaves and fry briefly till the radish is limp.

9. Add the radish tops together with the radishes and serve right away.

Paleo Barbeque pottage

Ingredients

- Onion, 1, diced

- Butter, 3 tablespoons

- Fat from bacon, 3teaspoons

- Garlic, 4 cloves, chopped

- Canned tomato sauce, 2 (12 ounce each)

- Worcestershire sauce, 2 teaspoons

- Liquid smoke, (mesquite or hickory flavor), 4 teaspoons

- Tabasco sauce, 2 teaspoons

- Gravy flavoring (such as Gravy Master or Kitchen Bouquet), 1 teaspoon

- Just like sugar sweetener, 8 packets

- Splenda, 2 packets

- Cider vinegar, 1 cup

- Salt, 1 teaspoon

- Pepper, ½ teaspoon

Preparation

1. Briefly fry the garlic and onion in the bacon fat and butter till they are tender.

2. Put the remaining ingredients and simmer, with the lid removed, at low heat for around 40 minutes.

3. Use an immersion blender or a food processor to puree the mixture in order to make the sauce smooth.

4. It will fill around 4 cups.

Carne Asada In Crock Pot

Ingredients

- Chuck roast, 1 pound

- Juice extracted from 1/2 orange

- Juice extracted from 1 lime

- Olive oil (extra virgin), ½ cup

- Fresh cilantro (diced), ½ cup

- Ground red pepper, ½ teaspoon

- Garlic, 2 cloves, diced

- Coconut sugar (not compulsory), ½ teaspoon

- Coriander, ½ teaspoon

- Oregano, 1 teaspoon

- Cumin, ½ teaspoon

- Sea salt, 1 teaspoon

- Half of a big-sized shallot, diced

Preparation

1. Under cold water, rinse the chuck roast before patting it dry. Keep the chuck roast aside and allow it to stand for about 25 minutes.

2. Put all the other ingredients in a food processor and grind to mix.

3. Generously coat the crock pot with asada marinade before putting the chuck roast.

4. In order to encourage the even heating of the meat (and avoid scorching), pour half cup of filtered water into the crock pot. Then set oven to high and allow it to cook for about 4 hours 45 minutes, making sure you flip its other side hourly.

5. Bring down the crock pot, remove the chuck and allow it to cool off for about 15 minutes.

6. The meat should be sliced meat across the grain and juice from crock pot spooned over.

Mayonnaise Veggie Coleslaw

Ingredients

- Tomatoes (ripe) cut into 1-inch sized cuts

- Haas Avocado (fairly ripe), diced into cubes

- Mayonnaise, 1 tablespoon

- Chopped onion, 1 ounce or onion powder, ½ teaspoon

- Salt

Preparation

1. Mix all the ingredients in a bowl, and stir properly.

2. Serve right away, or transfer to a container that can be sealed, then refrigerate.

Asian Beef And Broccoli Slaw

Ingredients

- ½ bag of broccoli slaw

- 1 lb ground beef

- 2 tablespoon organic tamari gluten free soy or coconut aminos

- 1 medium onion, chopped

- 1 pack mushrooms

- 1 tablespoon sherry

- 2 garlic cloves, chopped

- ½ tablespoon Coconut oil

- Handful of spinach

- ½ teaspoon Celtic salt dash of pepper

Preparation

1. Pour the coconut oil into a big cooking pan. Heat on high heat and then stir in the mushrooms. After about 4 to 5 minutes, stir in the onions, followed by the broccoli slaw. Combine them all together while it's cooking and then leave to stand for a couple of minutes.

2. Boil the meat in another big cooking pan until it turns brown. Next pour it into the pan holding the broccoli slaw mixture, stir in the Tamari or coconut aminos, spinach, pepper, salt and sherry.

3. Leave to simmer on low heat for a couple of minutes so the flavors can scent properly. Serve.

Roasted Paprika with Zucchini Chips

Ingredients

- 2 average-sized zucchini

- 1 teaspoon of salt

- 3 teaspoons of extra virgin olive oil

- Smoked paprika, 2 teaspoons

- Pepper (ground), 1 teaspoon

Preparation

1. Use a sharp knife or mandolin slicer to slash the zucchini across its length into thick cuts of 1/3 inch length.

2. Arrange the zucchini into a sieve or colander in layers, and then sprinkle each layer with a tiny amount of salt. Then allow it to drain for about 65 minutes.

3. Use parchment paper to line the inside of a baking sheet, and then heat oven to about 245F.Apply 2 teaspoons of oil on the parchment.

4. Use a paper towel to gently stroke the zucchini slices dry before placing them on a ready-made baking sheet. Apply some remaining oil to the zucchini tops and add a sprinkling of ground pepper and paprika.

5. Bake for about 50 minutes, switch the oven off and allow the chips remain enclosed till they are crispy. This would take about 70 minutes.

Bacon and Veggies

Ingredients

- Raw spinach, 12 ounces

- White onion (diced), 1/3 cup

- Shallot (diced), 1/3 cup

- Sliced raw bacon, 1/3 pound

- Butter, 3 tablespoons

Preparation

1. Cross slice the bacon into little narrow pieces.

2. Put some butter in a big skillet.

3. Put the shallots, bacon and diced onion. Fry for around 20-30 minutes or till bacon is cooked and the onions have turned brown.

4. Put in the spinach leaves.

5. Fry briefly at average heat with intermittent stirring, ensuring that you flip the leaves to enable contact of the top leaves with the hot skillet, while the pile cooks down. This also aids in combining the onions and the bacon.

6. Secure the lid of the skillet and allow the spinach mixture to steam for around 7 minutes. Stir repeatedly till the spinach is cooked and limp.

Bacon And Egg Zucchini Squash

Ingredients

- 5 slices boiled bacon, hopped and shredded

- 2 cups zucchini squash, crushed

- 8 eggs

- 1 teaspoon sea salt

- 2 tablespoon coconut flour or golden flax meal

- 3 cloves garlic, skinned and chopped

- 2 eggs, whisked

- ½ teaspoon black pepper

- ¾ cup cheese, shredded, optional

Preparation

1. Preheat the oven to 400 degrees, and rub nonstick spray on a large-sized muffin pan.

2. Use a grater or food processor to puree the zucchini until smooth. Pour the grated zucchini into a cheese cloth or layered paper towels and fold it up and drain out the surplus water. Endeavour to squeeze out as much moisture as possible.

3. Place the drained, squeezed zucchini into a big mixing bowl and stir in the pepper, minced garlic, coconut flour, salt, crushed cheese and the 2 whisked eggs. Combine all together.

4. Pour about 2 tablespoons of the zucchini mixture into the muffin pan cups. Dent a space in the center of each zucchini cup using a spoon.

5. Bake the zucchini cups alone for about 10-12 minutes.

6. Take out from the oven and top each zucchini with a little shredded bacon, and then crack an egg into each zucchini nest.

7. Bake for about 20 minutes or until the egg is done as you like. Take out of the oven, and leave to cool. Loosen the nests from the muffin cup using a butter knife.

Barbecued Lemon-spiced Sardines

Ingredients

- 4 whole large sardines

- 1¼ teaspoon marjoram

- 1½ tablespoon grass-fed ghee or butter, dissolved

- 2 springs fresh sliced thyme

- Juice of a lemon

- 1 garlic cloves, thinly sliced

- cracked black pepper

- Coarse salt

Preparation

1. Preheat the grill to very high heat.

2. Mix together the ghee and herbs in a medium-sized mixing bowl using a fork.

3. Coat the outside and inside of the sardines with the herb and ghee mixture.

4. Season the outside of the sardines with cracked black pepper and coarse salt.

5. Place the sardines on the grill basket and grill each side on high heat for about 2 to 3 minutes or until it turns crispy.

6. Take sardines out of the grill and serve with lemon juice.

Homemade Chicken And Veggie Sauce

Ingredients

- Organic chicken (dark meat); legs or thighs, 2 pounds

- Kosher salt, 1 teaspoon

- 1 big onion, cut into four parts

- Celery, 1 stalk, chopped

- 2 big carrot, with peel removed, diced

- Garlic, 1clove, peeled

- Cold water, 2 quarts

- Thyme leaves (dried), ½ teaspoon

- Parsley (dried), ½ teaspoon

- 1 bay leaf

- 4 big peppercorns

Preparation

1. Firstly heat the oven to 380F

2. Put the chicken in a big roasting pan or Dutch oven measuring 6.5 quarts. Add a sprinkling of salt then put the vegetables.

3. Place it on the oven's center rack and roast for almost 40 minutes.

4. Bring down from the oven and put on the stove burner.

5. Add the seasoning then pour some water into the pot. Simmer at average-low heat, being cautious to prevent the mixture from coming to full boil. As soon as it is simmering, remove any impurities or foam that might collect on the surface of the water and decrease the heat to low.

6. Set the oven to low heat and carefully simmer the mixture for almost 4 hours, removing any impurities or foam that may collect at the top.

7. Bring stockpot down from heat and allow it to cool for about 50-60 minutes.

8. Use a fine strainer to sieve the before broth before transferring to containers safe for storing food.

9. Throw away the strained solids.

10. Refrigerate overnight, and then remove the fat.

11. Use right away or refrigerate to store for future use.

Turkey And Avocado Rolls

Ingredients

- Softened cream cheese, 4 ounces

- Haas Avocado (ripe, average size), ½, spooned from the shell and diced

- Mayonnaise, 1 teaspoon

- Diced garlic clove, ¼ teaspoon; or granulated garlic, 1/8 teaspoon

- Finely diced onion, 1 ounce; or powdered onion, 1/8 teaspoon

- Salt

- Smoked turkey (thinly sliced), ½ pound

Preparation

1. Mix the cream cheese till it is of a smooth consistence with the help.

2. Put the rest of the ingredients and for an extra two minutes till the mixture is smooth.

3. Spread out turkey slices on paper towels and stroke lightly to dry if necessary.

4. Gently apply a thin layer of avocado cheese mixture on the whole turkey.

5. Like you would a jelly roll, roll the turkey slice, beginning from one end.

6. Serve right away, or refrigerate in a container that can be sealed.

Bacon and Egg Salad

Ingredients

- Eggs, 4

- Mayonnaise, 1 tablespoon

- Dijon mustard, ½ teaspoon

- Lemon juice, ½ teaspoon

- Lite salt, ½ teaspoon (to obtain potassium)

- Pepper and kosher salt to taste

Preparation

In an average-sized saucepan, gently put the eggs. Pour some cold water till the eggs are immersed up to around one inch. Allow to boil for about twelve minutes. Bring down from heat and allow it to cool. Under running cold water, peel the eggs. Put the eggs in a magic bullet or a food processor or and pulse till it is minced. Add the lemon juice, mustard, mayonnaise, pepper and salt. Taste and, as necessary, make adjustments. Serve with a wrapping of bacon and lettuce leaves if you like (not compulsory).

One-Skillet Buttery Bacon And Shrimp

Ingredients

- 5 oz. raw peeled shrimp

- 6 slices organic uncured bacon

- 5 oz. smoked salmon

- 1¼ cup chopped mushrooms

- 1 cup heavy whipping cream or coconut cream for a dairy-free option

- Freshly grated black pepper

- 1 dash of Celtic Sea Salt

Preparation

1. Slice the bacon in 1-inch bits.

2. Heat a cast iron skillet over a medium flame and pour the bacon into it.

3. Once the bacon is done but not yet crispy, stir in the chopped mushrooms and boil for about 5 minutes.

4. Stir in the chopped smoked salmon, and boil for another 2 to 3 minutes.

5. Pour in the shrimp and sauté' on a high heat for about 2 minutes.

6. Next stir in the cream and the salt, reduce the heat and simmer for another minute, or until the cream is as thick as preferred.

7. Serve at once.

8. You can serve with zucchini noodles or shirataki.

Baked Fiber Chops

Ingredients

- 4:1 Ratio

- Flax meal, 8g

- Psyllium husks (whole), 8g

- Baking powder, ½ gram

- Baking soda, ½ gram

- Salt, ¼ teaspoon

- Raw egg, 35g, mixed thoroughly

- Safflower or sunflower oil, 25g

- Cider vinegar, 2g

Preparation

1. Firstly heat oven to 290F

2. Combine the vinegar, oil and eggs thoroughly.

3. Put in the psyllium husks, baking soda, flax meal, salt and baking powder to the egg mixture. Stir with a spatula to thoroughly combine the ingredients.

4. Upon combination of the ingredients, allow the dough to sit for 4 minutes. They dough will give off a very wet appearance, but as it rests, the dough will increase in stiffness up to the consistency of oatmeal that is very stiff.

5. Use parchment paper to line one baking sheet. Split the dough evenly into 4 parts.

6. To avoid sticking, shape the dough however you like with wet hands. Bake on the baking sheet for half an hour.

7. Serve.

Creamy Vegetable Chops

Ingredients

- Softened cream cheese, 12 ounces

- Heavy cream, 1 cup

- Sour cream, 1 cup

- Onion, (diced), ½ cup

- Diced paprika, ½ cup

- Celery (diced), ½ cup

- Carrot (diced), ½ cup

- Broccoli (chopped), ½ cup

- Salt, 2 teaspoons

- Seasoned salt, 1 teaspoon

Preparation

1. Firstly whisk the cream cheese till it is fluffy.

2. Pour in the sour cream and cream. Put in the rest of the ingredients and stir properly.

3. Scoop spoonfuls into small tart crusts that have been pre-baked.

4. Bake for about 15 minutes at 345F or till it starts to bubble.

Lemon-Spiced Cheesecake

Ingredient

- Softened cheese cream, 4 ounces

- Heavy cream, 1 ounce

- Stevia Glycerite, ½ teaspoon

- Splenda or other low carb sweetener (liquid or powdered)

- Lemon juice, ½ tablespoon

- Vanilla flavoring, ½ teaspoon

Preparation

Combine all ingredients together and whip till it is as thick as a pudding. Serve small quantities into little serving cups and store in a fridge till it sets.

Ham And Alfredo Stew

Ingredient

- Butter, 2 tablespoons

- Baked ham, diced, ½ cup

- Heavy cream, ½ cup

- Egg yolk from 1 big egg

- Asiago cheese (freshly grated), 1 cup

- Granulated garlic, ¼ teaspoon

- White pepper, ¼ teaspoon

- Any of basil, parsley or thyme, ½ teaspoon (not compulsory)

- Pepper and salt

Preparation

1. Melt butter in an average-sized saucepan at average-high heat.

2. Put the ham and fry briefly for almost 2 minutes.

3. Add the egg yolk and cream and mix, then cook for an additional 4-5 minutes, lowering the heat to average low.

4. Put grated cheese and granulated garlic and mix. Simmer for around 4 minutes, with intermittent stirring.

5. Add to chicken or vegetable dish of your choice.

6. Serve at once!

Italian Meat And Tomato Sauce

Ingredients

- 1 can green olives

- 1 pack grass-fed shredded beef

- 1 can black olives

- 6 pork or chicken sausages

- 2 tablespoons fat

- 7 tomatoes, chopped

- 1 pack shredded mushrooms

- 2 small onion, chopped

- 1 yellow bell pepper, chopped

- 2 tablespoon dried basil

- 2 green bell pepper, chopped

- 2 tablespoon Italian Seasoning

- 3 cloves garlic, grated

- Sea salt and pepper to taste

Preparation

1. Heat a big pot over medium-high heat. Pour in the fat and allow it to dissolve.

2. Pour in the ground beef and cook.

3. Unwrap the sausages from their casings and stir the meat into the ground beef.

4. Boil until the ground beef is no longer pink.

5. Once the meat is cooked, chop the tomatoes and stir it into the pot when the beef is fully done.

6. Simmer the meat and tomatoes together for a couple of minutes, or until the tomatoes begin to dissolve.

7. As the tomatoes boil, dice the onion and stir into the pot when the tomatoes are done, stir properly.

8. Boil the sauce for a couple of minutes more.

9. Stir in the diced mushrooms and mix thoroughly.

10. Dice both bell peppers and when the mushrooms are fairly done stir it into the pot.

11. Stir in the garlic and seasonings as well. Leave to simmer for roughly 15 minutes.

12. pour in the olives and leave to boil for an additional 12 to 15 minutes, or until the sauce becomes as thick as preferred.

13. Serve.

Barbecued Cardoons And Lamb Chops

Ingredients

LAMB CHOPS

- 3 medium cloves organic garlic

- 3 lamb shoulder chops

- Celtic sea salt

- 2½ tablespoons olive oil

- 2 sprig fresh rosemary

CARDOONS

- 1 bunch cardoons, washed, skinned, diced to 4-inch lengths

- Celtic sea salt

Preparation

LAMB CHOPS

1. Using a small food processor, combine the oil, rosemary, garlic, and salt together.

2. Remove the lamb chops from the refrigerator to defrost.

3. Arrange the chops in a small plate and coat with the oil mixture.

4. Cover it and allow to stand for roughly 30 minutes or until they attain room temperature.

5. Heat a cast iron skillet on medium heat until a droplet of water bounces off when dropped on it.

6. Arrange the chops inside the skillet and grill each side for approximately 5 minutes or until the internal temperature of 125 degrees is attained.

7. Allow the chops to cool for about 5 minutes in a warm covered plate before serving.

CARDOONS

8. Boil a quart of water in a small pot.

9. Season with a dash of sea salt.

10. pour in the cardoons and boil for around 15 to 20 minutes or until it shreds when pierced with a fork.

11. Drain properly.

12. While the lamb chops are cooling, fry the cardoons using the same cast iron skillet, still holding the cooking juices from the lamb chops.

13. Serve together while it is still hot.

Chocolate Protein Shake

Ingredients

- Almond milk (unsweetened), 8 ounces

- Heavy cream, 2 ounces

- Powdered Chocolate Whey Isolate (Jay Robb brand), 1 scoop

- Sugar Free Strawberry Syrup (DaVinci brand), ½ tablespoon

- Crushed ice, ¼ cup (not compulsory)

Preparation

Blend all the ingredients in a blender till it is smooth.

Roasted Lemon-Spiced Asparagus

Ingredients

- 1-pound asparagus (with tough ends cut off), 2 bunches

- Gluten-free Dijon mustard, 2 teaspoons

- Olive oil (extra virgin), 4 tablespoons

- Lemon, 2

- Fresh herbs (diced), e.g. chives, tarragon, parsley, 2 tablespoons

- Sea salt to taste

- Fat for roasting, 4 tablespoons

Preparation

1. Firstly heat the oven to 440F.

2. Use the fat you prefer to toss the asparagus, and then spread it on a baking sheet. (You may line the baking sheet with parchment if you like)

3. As soon as oven is hot, roast the asparagus for about 15-22 minutes, contingent on the thickness of the asparagus.

4. Prepare the lemon vinaigrette in the meantime.

5. Peel the lemon, and then proceed to squeeze 2 tablespoons of the juice into a little bowl. Then keep the peels on one side.

6. Pour the olive oil, mustard and herbs and mix using a whisk.

7. As soon the asparagus is soft and a little caramel in color, add a sprinkling of sea salt and transfer to a serving platter.

8. Use the zest to garnish and pour the vinaigrette on it.

9. You can serve either cold, at room temperature or hot.

Buffalo Chicken And Veggie Coleslaw

Ingredients

- 4 tablespoon hot sauce

- 4 medium red or yellow bell peppers or a few handfuls of small sweet peppers

- 6 pieces of chicken thighs or breasts, grilled or baked, then cooled

- Lots of diced green onions

- 3 tablespoon Greek yogurt

- Dash of celery salt

- 1½ teaspoon garlic powder

- **Optional:** blue cheese, garnished on top, diced celery

Preparation

Combine all the ingredients together in a big mixing bowl. Mix properly and serve on top of greens.

Barbecued Salmon With Veggie Salsa

Ingredients

SALMON:

• Pinch of salt and freshly grated black pepper

• 1 pound wild sockeye or salmon fillet, boneless

SALSA:

• 3 tablespoons cilantro leaves, finely diced

• 1 English cucumber, skinned, seeded and thinly diced

• 2 tablespoon mint leaves, thinly diced

• 1 cup sweet onion, thinly sliced

• 1 ½ teaspoon avocado oil or olive oil

• 1 whole Serrano chili, remove stem and thinly sliced

• 1 lime, juiced

• ¼ teaspoon freshly grated black pepper

• ¼ teaspoon kosher salt

Preparation

1. Spice the salmon with the kosher salt and freshly grated black pepper. Leave aside.

2. Skin the cucumber and slice into fine pieces.

3. Combine in a bowl together with the cilantro, diced onion, Serrano chili and mint. Pour in the lime juice, oil, pepper and salt. Flip to coat and refrigerate until it's ready to be served.

4. Grill the salmon fillet with a hickory board. If placing the salmon directly on top of the grill, rub oil on the skin and boil the skin side down with lid covered.

5. Serve.

Marinated Oven-Baked Salmon

Ingredients

- Garlic (diced), 1 clove

- Light olive oil, 3 tablespoons

- Basil (dried), ½ teaspoon

- Salt, ½ teaspoon

- Black pepper (ground), ½ teaspoon

- Lemon juice, ½ tablespoon

- Fresh parsley (diced), ½ tablespoon

- Salmon fillets, 1 (3 ounces)

Preparation

1. Make marinade in an average-sized glass bowl by mixing the parsley, garlic, lemon juice, light olive oil, salt, basil, and pepper. Use the marinade to cover the salmon fillets, and then put it in an average-sized glass baking dish. Marinate in the refrigerator around 60 minutes, with periodical stirring.

2. Heat the oven to 375F. Cover the fillets with marinade; put them in aluminum foil, then seal. Put the sealed salmon inside the glass dish using a fork, and bake for 30 to 40 minutes, or till it is flaky.

Chocolate Chip Mini Muffins

Ingredients

- Almond flour, 1 cup

- Erythritol, ½ cup

- Baking soda, ¼ cup

- Salt, ¼ teaspoon

- Xanthan gum, ¼ teaspoon

- 1 big egg to be slightly beaten

- Sour cream, ½ cup

- Melted and fairly cooled butter, 1 tablespoon

- Stevia glycerite, 1 teaspoon

- Caramel dip (Walden Farms SF brand), ¼ cup

- Any of diced ChocoPerfection, Lilly's chocolate chips or Enjoy Life Semi-sweet chocolate chips, ½ cup

Preparation

1. Firstly heat oven to 340F and use paper liners to line 45 mini-muffin cups.

2. Mix the baking soda, almond flour, erythritol, xanthan gum and salt together in an average-sized bowl.

3. Beat the eggs slightly in a smaller bowl before putting the cooled butter, stevia and sour cream.

4. Combine the almond flour and the liquid mixture then mix thoroughly.

5. Fill individual muffin cups to around ¾ of their capacity.

6. Bake for about 18-23 minutes, or till the muffin tops are springy-firm to the touch and fairly brown in colour.

7. Remove and allow it to cool. Cooling makes it less difficult to remove the paper.

8. Store them in a sealed container and refrigerate.

Vegan Chocolate Easter Eggs

Ingredients

Paleo Easter Eggs

- 4 tablespoon coconut cream

- 3 oz unsweetened coconut, hopped

- 1 teaspoon vanilla

- 3 oz. coconut oil, dissolved

- 2 tablespoon granulated stevia, or sweetener, to taste

Chocolate Coating

- 5 teaspoon cocoa powder

- 2.5 oz. coconut oil, dissolved

- 2 ½ teaspoon granulated stevia, or sweetener, to taste

Preparation

Paleo Easter Eggs

1. Combine all the ingredients in a medium-sized bowl.

2. Place in Refrigerator until hard enough to fold into egg shapes.

3. Fold small quantities into egg shapes and refrigerate once more to harden wholly.

Chocolate Coating

1. Combine all the ingredients in a medium-sized mixing bowl.

2. Put one Paleo Easter Egg inside the chocolate coating one at a time. Flip the egg until fully covered using a spoon.

3. Put the chocolate-coated eggs on a dish.

4. Place in the refrigerator until the chocolate coating is fully set.

Swiss Meatball Cookies

Ingredients

- White onions (diced), 2 ounces

- Butter, ½ tablespoon

- Swiss cheese, 2 ounces

- Whole milk ricotta cheese (cold), ½ cup

- 1 big egg (cold)

- Nutmeg powder, 1 teaspoon

- Allspice, 1 teaspoon

- Sea salt, 1teaspoon

- Black pepper (freshly ground), half teaspoon

- 90% lean ground beef, ½ pound

Preparation

1. Briefly fry the onions in butter till they are semi-transparent, then bring it down and allow cool for about 15 minutes.

2. With the onions cooling, chop the Swiss cheese, and then finely dice the shreds using a food processor. Keep it aside.

3. Combine egg and ricotta cheese inside a mixing bowl.

4. Put the pepper, salt and spices then mix.

5. Put Swiss cheese and onions and stir till it is smooth.

6. Introduce the beef and stir till all ingredients form stick-free dough.

7. Split the meat mixture into 12 pieces each size being one ounce.

8. Make individual pieces into a ball shape.

9. Put meatballs on a cookie sheet and proceed to bake at 345F till it is brown and properly cooked.

Baked Meat Bagel

Ingredients

- 2 onions, minced

- 2 tablespoons of bacon fat/grass fed ghee/butter etc.

- Pork (ground), 3 pounds

- 3 big eggs

- Tomato sauce, 1 cup

- Paprika, 2 teaspoons

- Salt, 2 teaspoons

- Pepper (ground), 1 teaspoon

Preparation

1. Firstly heat the oven to 400F. Then use parchment paper to line the inside of a baking dish.

2. After step 1, fry the onions over average heat with cooking fat of your choice (such as grass fed ghee, butter etc.). Sauté till it is semi-transparent. Ensure that the onions cool off before you add them to the meat.

3. Mix the ingredients and the cooked onions in a bowl. Mix properly in order to distribute spices equally.

4. The meat should then be split into 8 parts. Manually roll a part of the meat into a round shape, and then make a piercing at the centre. Flatten the meat a little bit in order to get the shapes of a bagel.

5. Put the bagel-shaped meat inside the dish and replicate step 4 above with the other parts of the meat.

6. Bake for about 45 minutes or till the meat is tender.

7. Remove the meat bagels and allow them to cool down. Slice the meat bagel like you would a normal bagel. Use toppings such as lettuce, onions, tomato slice etc. to fill the meat bagels.

Fried Sardine With Turnip Au Roquefort

Ingredients

- Roquefort cheese, 10g

- Sardine, 15g

- Turnip, 40g

- Mayonnaise, 25g

Preparation

1. Peel the turnip, dice it and boil it.

2. Combine the mayonnaise and the turnip, and spread with the Roquefort cheese. Set aside.

3. Fry the sardines and later on, serve the turnip with Roquefort cheese.

Paleo Crock-Pot Minced Pork

Ingredients

- 1 6oz - 8oz can organic tomato paste

- 2 lbs pork loin

- 2½ tablespoons coconut oil

- 3 tablespoons lemon juice

- 2 jalapeno pepper, seeded

- 2 small onion, diced

- 3 teaspoon chili powder

- 3 garlic cloves, chopped

- 1¼ teaspoon thyme

- 1½ teaspoon cumin

- ¾ teaspoon paprika

- 1 teaspoon cayenne pepper

Preparation

1. Mix together all ingredients in a crock pot.

2. Heat the crock pot on low heat and boil for about 5 hours.

3. When it is properly done, use two forks to tear up the pork.

4. Serve.

Cheesy Salmon And Shrimp Sauce

Ingredients

• Cream cheese, 3 ounces

• Mayonnaise (full fat), 1.5 ounces

• Sea salt, ½ teaspoon

• Black pepper, ¼ teaspoon

• Lemon juice, ½ teaspoon

• Dried dill, ¼ teaspoon

• Pink salmon (boneless and skinless, canned), 3 ounces

• Shrimp (steamed or boiled), 2 ounces

Preparation

1. Place the cream cheese in a glass bowl, and then microwave it for just under 45 seconds to soften it. Bring down from the microwave, add mayonnaise, and mix till it is smooth. Add in the lemon juice and spices mix.

2. Put the shrimp and salmon and shrimp in a food processor bowl that has an S-blade. Put the cream cheese mixture and blend for around 25 - 500 seconds to an even consistency. You may consume right away or serve later.

Lamb with Rhubarb Stew

Ingredients

- Olive oil (or beef tallow), 4 tablespoons

- 2 big onions, diced

- Celery, 2 stalks (diced)

- 2 pounds or 1kg leg of boneless lamb,(cut to bite-sized pieces)

- Garlic, 3 cloves

- Butter, 3 tablespoons

- Turmeric, 1 teaspoon

- Honey (or brown sugar), 2 teaspoons

- Zest and juice from 1 lemon,

- Salt, 2 teaspoons

- White pepper, 1 teaspoon

- Fresh mint, 40g, diced

- Flat-leaf parsley, 200g or 4 cups or 150 g, diced

- Chicken stock, 1litre or 4 cups

- Dried mint, 1 teaspoon

- Rhubarb, 1 kg or 2 pounds, chopped diagonally into 3 inch pieces

- 1 teaspoon of ground saffron thread dissolved in 3-4 tablespoons of hot water

Preparation

1. Warm your preferred fat in a stew pot over average to high heat, then fry meat till it turns brown.

2. After step 1 above, turn the heat down to average-low, take away the meat, then put the celery and onions, making sure to scrap the brown bits from the base of the pan. Allow to cook for about seven minutes or till the onions are fairly brown and clear.

3. Put back the meat together with the turmeric, lemon, garlic, sugar, lemon zest (keep the juice for subsequent use), butter, and fresh herbs, pepper and salt. Allow to cook for around seven minutes before adding chicken stock and the dried mint.

4. Open the cover slightly and boil slowly at low heat for about 60 minutes, stirring occasionally as it is cooking.

5. Pour the saffron liquid and the diced rhubarb, and allow it to cook for about 25 minutes, this time without stirring.

6. Taste and put additional lemon juice as necessary or even a little extra honey or sugar.

7. Bring down and serve.

Creamy Bacon With Kale

Ingredients

- Kale leaves, ½ of a big bunch

- Onion, diced, ½ cup

- Garlic cloves, 2

- Raw bacon (3-4 slices) or bacon grease, 1 tablespoon

- Butter, 1 tablespoon

Preparation

1. Put diced raw bacon (or bacon grease) and butter in a big skillet.

2. Put the diced garlic and onion. Fry briefly for a few minutes or till the bacon has started to cook or the onions are tender.

3. Put in the kale leaves.

4. Fry briefly at average heat, with intermittent stirring, ensuring that the leaves are flipped so that all parts come in contact with the hot skillet, while the pile cooks. This move also helps in combining the onions and bacon.

5. Cook kale leaves till they are soft as desired. This should last more or less depending on how soft you want it to be and the heat temperature.

Oven-Baked Cheddar Biscuits

Ingredients

Wet Ingredients

- 5 eggs

- ½ cup tallow, dissolved

- 2 ½ teaspoons apple cider vinegar

Dry Ingredients

- 1 teaspoon gluten-free baking powder

- 2 cups coarsely powdered almond flour

- ½ teaspoon Himalayan rock salt

- 1 teaspoon onion powder

Extras

- 2 ½ tablespoon shredded jalapenos, optional

- 1 cup Daiya dairy-free cheddar cheese, chopped

Preparation

1. Preheat the oven to 400 degrees and line silicone baking sheet or parchment paper inside a baking sheet. Leave to stand.

2. Mix together all the wet ingredients in a big mixing bowl and stir together. Set aside.

3. Pour all dry ingredients into a small mixing bowl, crush together until blended. Pour the dry ingredients into the wet one and whisk until combined.

4. Pour in the dairy-free cheddar cheese and shredded jalapenos.

5. Divide the batter into 8 patties on the prepared baking sheet. When arranged on the sheet, you're your hands to shape lightly.

6. Place in a preheated oven and bake for about 15 minutes, or until it turns brown. Take out of the oven and allow it to cool on the baking sheet.

7. Place in a sealed container and keep in the fridge for about 3 days, or in the freezer for upwards of 2 months.

Chips With Mint Pudding

Ingredients

Chips

- 1 cup coconut oil, dissolved

- 4 drops of stevia

- 1½ tablespoon cacao powder

Pudding

- 1¼ teaspoon peppermint oil

- 1 (15 oz.) canned full fat coconut milk

- 12 drops of Protocol Stevia

- 2 medium avocado, pitted

Preparation

1. To prepare the chips, combine the ingredients in a small bowl and stir with a fork or whisk until smooth.

2. Transfer into an oiled or parchment paper-lined small flat container and store in the fridge for about an hour until well set.

3. Take it out of the freezer and using a knife, slice it into coarse chips.

4. To prepare the pudding, combine all the ingredients in the blender and squash until it becomes smooth.

5. Pour in the chips and then store in the refrigerator to chill for about an hour.

Easy Buttery Egg Salad

Ingredients

- 8 large eggs

- Mayonnaise, ¼ cup

- Melted butter, 1 tablespoon

- Ground mustard, ¼ cup

- White onion (diced), ¼ cup

- Black pepper, ½ teaspoon

- Salt, ½ teaspoon

Preparation

1. In a big pot, pour cold water to the brim, and then gently place the eggs. Boil the water till it is very hot, and then cook the eggs for about 15 minutes.

2. Bring the pot down and drain the water. Allow the eggs to remain in the pot then refill the pot with cold water.

3. Allow the eggs to cool to about 4-5 minutes.

4. Take out the eggs, dry and peel them.

5. Cut the peeled eggs into equal pieces of 1/3 inch each. You may use an egg slicer.

6. Put the rest of the ingredients and stir properly. Store in a refrigerator till it is time to serve.

Creamy Chocolate Avocado Shake

Ingredients

- 5 teaspoon honey

- 2 ripe avocadoes

- 3 tablespoon unsweetened almond or coconut milk

- 4 tablespoon cocoa powder

- 1¼ teaspoon vanilla

Preparation

1. Pour the entire ingredients into a food processor, or blender and blend together.

2. Blend until it becomes smooth and creamy.

3. Serve.

Chocolate Cheesecake Chips

Ingredient

- Dissolved cream cheese, 4 ounces

- Heavy cream, 1 ounce

- Stevia Glycerite, ½ teaspoon

- Splenda (packet) or other low carb sweetener (liquid or powdered)

- Chocolate chips (Enjoy Life Mini brand), ½ ounce

Preparation

Combine the ingredients (excluding the chips) and mix till it has the consistency of a pudding. Gently add chocolate chips in folds. Scoop into serving cups of small size and store in a refrigerator till it sets.

Spicy Meaty Tacos

Ingredients

- Butter, 1 tablespoon

- ½ yellow onion, diced,

- Garlic, 2 cloves, diced

- Ground beef, ½ pound

- Canned green chillies, 2 ounces

- Ground cumin, 1 teaspoon

- Chilli powder, 1 teaspoon

- Ground coriander, ½ teaspoon

- Sour cream, ¼ cup

- Grated cheddar cheese or Monterey Jack cheese, 2 cups

Preparation

1. Fry onions briefly in a medium skillet till they are tender.

2. Put in the ground beef and fry till they turn brown and are thoroughly cooked.

3. Put the spices and chilies then simmer for about 4 minutes.

4. Reduce the heat then add cheese and sour cream.

5. Set heat to low and simmer for around 12 minutes, with intermittent stirring to combine the ingredients.

6. Scoop a spoonful into each small low carb pie crusts that have been pre-baked.

7. Set oven to 340F and bake till it is foaming. This would take around 15 minutes.

8. Serve.

Cup-Baked Ham And Eggs

Ingredients

• 2 slices Ham or Turkey

• 2 Eggs

• Scallions, Optional

Preparation

1. Preheat the oven to about 400 degrees.

2. Rub nonstick spray on the Muffin or Cupcake Pan.

3. Place 1 or 2 slices of ham into each muffin cup.

4. Depending on whether you prefer your eggs scrambled or not, you can break an egg into another cup and whisk it prior to pouring it into the ham cups. Add the diced mushrooms, spinach and scallions.

5. If you like you prefer the eggs whole, then crack the egg into a cup.

6. Garnish with a few pieces of sliced scallions, optional

7. Place the muffin pan inside the oven preheated to about 400°F and bake it for about 15 minutes or until the eggs are done to your taste.

Bacon with Spiced Mayonnaise

Ingredients

- 2 egg yolks (organic)

- Dijon mustard, 1 teaspoon

- Juice squeezed from fresh lemon or white wine vinegar, 2 teaspoons

- Ground pepper (fresh) and sea salt, 2 teaspoons

- Light olive oil (½ cup) mixed with liquid bacon fat (½ cup) in a glass measuring cup.

Preparation

1. Put the mustard, egg yolk and lemon juice inside a food processor's small bowl, then process to combine.

2. Ensure the olive oil or bacon fat is liquefied, but not necessarily hot.

3. While the machine is still running, pour the olive oil/bacon fat in a thin stream little by little till the combination begins to form an emulsion and get stiff. This would take around 3 minutes.

4. Should the mayonnaise become very thick, you can thin it by adding a teaspoon of hot water to it.

5. Taste and add more spices if need be.

Creamy Radish Browns

Ingredients

- 1½ tablespoon bacon grease or butter

- 1 tablespoon extra-virgin olive oil

- 2 medium green onions, diced

- 2 cups chopped radishes

- ¼ cup red onion, diced

- ¼ cup red bell pepper, seeded and diced

- 2½ tablespoons Italian parsley, shredded

- 2 jalapeno chili pepper, finely chopped with seeds

- Sea salt

- 1 clove garlic, skinned and thinly chopped

- Fresh powdered black pepper

Preparation

Mix together all the ingredients in a big, heavy skillet and heat over medium heat. Boil to the preferred doneness, stirring repeatedly. Serve.

Dirty Rice With Shrimp Chorizo

Ingredients

- 1 ½ lb medium shrimp, uncooked

- 3 tablespoon prepared salsa

- 1 lb raw chorizo

- 1 ½ tablespoon Cajun seasoning

- ¾ cup white wine

- 3 teaspoon garlic powder

- 1½ tablespoon butter

- 2 ½ cups cauliflower, riced

- ½ cup cilantro, diced

- ½ cup scallions, diced

- Salt and pepper to taste

- 1 tablespoon lime juice

Preparation

1. Separate the chorizo from the shell and boil in a big frying saucepan. Pour in the wine and cut by half. Stir in the shrimp, garlic powder, butter, salsa, and Cajun seasoning, to the saucepan. Boil for approximately 2 minutes. Stir in the cauliflower and boil for an additional 5 minutes until the shrimp is well done.

2. Turn off the heat and stir in the cilantro, scallions and lime juice.

3. Add the salt and pepper to taste and then serve.

Oven-Baked Ham And Mustard

Ingredients

- 2 smoked hams

- 1 cup mayonnaise

- 1¼ cup prepared mustard

- 3 tablespoon rosemary, diced

- 3 tablespoon garlic, chopped

- Freshly grated pepper

Preparation

1. Mix together all the ingredients in a medium-sized bowl.

2. Put the ham in a roasting pan with the fat side facing up. Drizzle sufficiently with the mustard mixture. Pour 1 cup of water into the pan and put in a 300 degree preheated oven. Leave uncovered and bake for around 15 minutes per lb.

3. Serve with your preferred low-carb side dishes.

Spicy Cheese Muffins

Ingredients

- Almond flour, 3 cups

- Baking soda, 1 teaspoon

- Salt, ½ teaspoon

- Thyme (dried), 1 teaspoon

- 4 eggs

- Sour cream, 2 cups

- Dissolved butter, ½ cup

- Colby jack or chopped cheddar, 2 cups

- Chopped Muenster, 1 cup

Preparation

1. Firstly heat the oven to about 400F. Put the cupcake papers singly in normal-sized muffin pan that can hold 12 muffins.

2. Combine the dry ingredients and almond flour and mix.

3. Whisk eggs gently in a different bowl, and then integrate the butter and sour cream.

4. Pour some liquid mixture to the almond flour mixture. You can thin the batter with one tablespoon of heavy cream or water if it is very thick.

5. Put in the cheese and mix till it is distributed equally.

6. Spoon mixture into muffin cups, filling each 3/4 full.

7. Set oven temperature to about 400F and bake for 7 minutes.

8. Reduce the temperature of the oven to about 350 degrees and bake for an additional 25 minutes or until it turns light brown. Allow it to cool and you can serve with butter.

Cheese and Vegetable Pesto

Ingredients

- Cilantro leaves (firmly packed), 2 cups

- Garlic, 3 big cloves, diced

- Black pepper and salt

- Virgin olive oil, 1/3 cup, split (less oil results in a denser pesto)

- Walnuts, ¼ cup

- Cashews (or macadamias or pecans), ¼ cup

- Roughly grated Parmesan, 2 ounces

- Softened butter, 1 tablespoon

Preparation

1. Fill food processor with cilantro and process several times to mince.

2. Put the pepper, salt, around 1/3 cup olive oil and garlic. Blend till the mixture is smooth.

3. Stop the processor motor, and then pour in the cheese, nuts and butter, then process until the mixture is smooth. Add extra olive oil to thin the mixture should it get very thick to mix.

4. Use a plastic wrap to cover the surface and refrigerate. The pesto can keep for up to 12 days, and can last about 6-7 months if frozen.

Oven-Roasted Paleo Shrimp Cocktail

Ingredients

- 1¼ tablespoon olive oil

- 1 pound raw shrimp, skinned, deveined, and defrosted

- Paleo cocktail sauce

- Fresh ground pepper and sea salt, to taste

- Lemon wedges

Preparation

1. Preheat the oven to 425 degrees.

2. Flip the shrimp in oil, pepper and salt and spread in a single layer on the baking sheet.

3. Roast, for about 5 to 10 minutes flipping once, until the shrimp is pink and done through.

4. Serve chilled with lemon wedges and paleo cocktail sauce.

Sautéed Chicken Tikka Masala

Ingredients

- 1 English Cucumber, finely chopped
- 1 (15-ounce) chopped Tomato
- 1 (14oz) Can Lite Coconut Milk
- 1½ tablespoon Garlic, chopped
- 2 small Onion, diced
- 1¼ tablespoon Garam Masala
- 3 tablespoons Tomato Paste
- 1¼ Cup Coconut Cream
- 1¼ teaspoon Cinnamon Powder
- 1¼ teaspoon powdered Coriander
- 2 Pounds Boneless, Skinless Chicken Thighs
- Black Pepper and Kosher Salt
- 1½ tablespoon Fresh Lemon Juice
- ½ Cup Fresh Cilantro Leaves
- 1¼ Tablespoon Olive Oil

Preparation

1. Pour olive oil into a 4- or 6-quart Dutch oven and stir-fry the chicken thighs until brown.

2. Mix together the cucumber, the lemon juice, cilantro, and ½ teaspoon each of pepper and salt in a small-sized mixing bowl. Replace cover and refrigerate for about 8 hours.

3. Take out the chicken from the Dutch oven, stir in the garlic and onion and stir-fry until the onion becomes translucent.

4. Pour the chicken back into the skillet, stir in the chopped tomatoes and juice, garam masala, coriander, salt, cinnamon, pepper and coconut milk.

5. When you have done all the above steps, stir in the tomato paste. Allow it to simmer for about half an hour or until the chicken is properly done and tender.

6. Before serving, pour the coconut cream into the chicken tikka masala.

White Chocolate Protein Shake

Ingredients

- Almond milk (unsweetened), 8 ounces

- Heavy cream, 2ounces

- Vanilla Whey Powder (Jay Robb Enterprises brand), 1 scoop

- Sugar Free White Chocolate syrup (Da Vinci brand), ½ tablespoon

- Crushed ice, ½ cup (not compulsory)

Preparation

Blend all ingredients in a food processor and blend till it's smooth.

Cinnamon Tea Eggs

Ingredients

- 7 cups of water

- 8 eggs

- 4 star anise

- 3 tablespoons sea salt

- 3 tea bags

- ½ tablespoon Szechuan peppercorns

- 1 tablespoons cinnamon

- ¾ cup tamari sauce or coconut aminos, optional

- ¾ teaspoon black pepper

Preparation

1. Boil the eggs in hot water till it becomes hard.

2. After boiling the eggs, allow it to cool and crack the shell without peeling it off the eggs.

3. Place the tea bags, cinnamon, salt, Szechuan pepper, black pepper, star anise, and tamari sauce inside a big pot.

4. Return the cracked eggs into the pot.

5. Pour 7 cups of water into the pot.

6. Cover and boil on a low heat.

7. After half an hour of boiling take out the tea bags.

8. Simmer for another 3-4 hours with the lid closed.

9. Allow the eggs to cool and peel off the shell.

Browned Taco And sauce

Ingredients

- Ground beef (without fat), 2 pounds

- Taco seasoning, 5 tablespoons

- Pico de gallo (or any salsa you prefer)

- Guacamole, 3 cups

- Iceberg lettuce (diced), 2 cups

- Black olives (minced), 2 cups

- Plantain chips to serve

Preparation

1. Place a big frying pan over average high heat and heat it. As soon as the pot is hot, add the taco seasoning and ground beef. Use a spoon to separate the meat and allow it to cook until it browns and has cooked thoroughly.

2. Before transferring the meat to a bowl drain it properly.

3. Arrange the cooked ground beef, chopped lettuce, guacamole, pico and sliced olives.

4. Take a trifle dish and start to layer. Disperse the ground beef on the bottom, the guacamole, followed by the pico de gallo. Add a sprinkling of minced black olives and diced lettuce. Partition the guacamole and ground beef pico into individual dishes then add a sprinkling of minced black olives and diced lettuce on each dish.

5. You can add this layer to any serving dish.

Vegan Cheesy Meatball Casserole

Ingredients

For the meatballs:

• 3 eggs

• 1 lb sweet or hot Italian sausage

• ½ cup crushed Parmesan cheese

• 1 lb shredded chuck or turkey

• 1½ tablespoon dried parsley

• ½ cup almond flour

• ½ teaspoon red pepper flakes

• 1¼ teaspoon kosher salt

• ¾ teaspoon onion powder

• ¾ teaspoon garlic powder

• ½ teaspoon dried oregano

For the casserole:

• 2 cups whole milk mozzarella cheese, minced

• 2½ cups keto marinara

• 1 cup whole milk ricotta cheese

Preparation

Preparing the meatballs:

1. Thoroughly mix together all the meatball ingredients inside a medium-sized mixing bowl. Roll into about 32, 1.5-inch meatballs. Arrange the meatballs on a baking sheet lined with parchment, and bake for about 15 minutes at 375 degrees.

Preparing the casserole:

2. Arrange the meatballs in a single layer inside a casserole dish. Drizzle half of the keto marinara sauce on top of the meatballs. Spread teaspoonfuls of the ricotta cheese generously over the casserole. Sprinkle the remaining half of the marinara sauce on top. Garnish the mozzarella cheese over the mixture. Bake for approximately half an hour at 375 degrees. Take the pan out of the oven and allow it cool for roughly 5 minutes before serving.

Almond Carrot Pancakes

Ingredients

Pancakes:

• 4 big eggs, whisked

• 1 cup almond flour

• ½ cup Swerve Sweetener or granulated erythritol

• 1 cup flax seed meal

• 1 ¼ teaspoon cinnamon

• 1 ½ teaspoon baking powder

• ½ cup avocado oil

• 1 ½ cup chopped carrot

• 2 tablespoon almond milk

• ½ cup pecans or walnuts, sliced

• Butter or oil for pan

• 2 ½ tablespoon diced raisins (optional)

• Dash of salt

Frosting:

• 1 tablespoon heavy cream

• 5 oz. cream cheese, melted

• 3 tablespoon ground Swerve Sweetener or ground erythritol

- 1 ½ tablespoon butter, dissolved

- 1 teaspoon vanilla extract

Preparation

1. Preparing the pancakes: mix together the cinnamon, erythtritol, flax seed meal, baking powder, and salt in a large mixing bowl.

2. Whisk in the oil, eggs and almond milk until properly mixed.

3. Add the diced nuts, raisins and carrots.

4. Heat a big pan over medium heat. Pour in 3 teaspoon of oil or butter and spin to cover the pan's bottom.

5. Using a little ¼ cup of batter for each of the pancakes, transfer batter onto the griddle and spread into roughly 4-inch circles.

6. Fry until the bottom turns brown and the top is stiff around the edges. Toss gently and keep on frying until the other side is brown as well. Transfer to a baking sheet or a plate and keep warm in the oven, while doing the same with the rest of the batter.

7. To prepare the frosting, whisk butter and cream cheese together in a mixing bowl until uniformly smooth. Stir in the ground erythritol, vanilla extract and the cream.

8. Serve the pancakes with a spoonful of frosting.

Blueberry Lemon-spiced Cakes

Ingredients

- Almond Flour, 4 cups

- Heavy cream, 2 cups

- 4 large eggs

- Butter (melted) ½ cup

- Stevia or splenda, 8 packets

- Baking soda, 1 teaspoon

- Lemon flavoring (or extract), 1 teaspoon

- Dried lemon peels, 1 teaspoon

- Salt, ½ teaspoon

- Blueberries (fresh), 2 ounces

Preparation

1. Firstly heat oven to 350F degrees. Put cupcake papers in single muffin holes of normal sized 12 count muffin pan. (You'll need about two pans).

2. Combine the cream and almond flour.

3. Put the eggs singly, and mix by stirring.

4. Put the baking soda, spices, flavoring, sweetener and butter, then mix.

5. Put in the blueberries and mix till it is distributed equally.

6. Half fill each cupcake and place in the pan.

7. Bake for around 15 minutes or till it turns light brown. Allow to cool, and then serve with butter.

Spinach and Apple Salad

Ingredients

- Young spinach leaves, washed, 5 cups

- Red onion, (sliced thinly), 1 cup

- Crushed blue cheese, 5tablespoons

- Apple (small sized), half, diced into cubes of 1/3 inches

Preparation

1. Split the spinach leaves among four plates of salad.

2. On each plate, spread thinly sliced red onion over the spinach.

3. Sprinkle the mixture on the apple.

4. Add a spoonful of your preferred choice of low carb salad dressing (e.g. Feta Vinagrette) and gently toss.

Quick Noodles With Beef Ragù

Ingredients

Beef ragu:

- 2 lb beef, grass-fed, chopped

- 1 ¼ tablespoon butter or ghee

- ½ cup red pesto

- Garlic or herb for extra flavor

- 1 teaspoon pink Himalayan salt to taste

- Small bunch fresh parsley

Noodles:

- 4 big zucchini, chopped using a vegetable spiralizer or julienne peeler

Preparation

1. Take the meat out of the fridge to slowly thaw.

2. Put the meat in a pan smeared with ghee and sauté for about 6 minutes until it turns evenly brown on all sides. Preserve some of the ghee for later use.

3. Stir in the red pesto and freshly diced parsley and simmer. When done turn off the heat and pour into a bowl.

4. Next, prepare the zucchini "noodles" using a spiralizer or julienne peeler. Slice the soft core of the zucchini and pour it into the zoodles.

5. Pour the noodles into the pan smeared with the rest of the ghee. Sauté for about 3 to 5 minutes. Switch off the heat, stir in the meat and combine thoroughly.

6. Serve.

Paleo Coconut Cookies

Ingredients

- Cocoa powder, 1 cup

- Organic eggs, 3

- Birch xylitol (organic) or raw honey or maple syrup, 1 cup; or extract of stevia powder, 3 teaspoons

- Melted coconut oil, 2 cups

- Full fat coconut milk (canned), 1 cup full fat

- Vanilla extract, 2 teaspoons

- Almond flour (preferably blanched), 2 cups

- Baking soda, 1 teaspoon

- Coconut (minced), 1 cup

- Walnuts (diced), 1 cup

Preparation

1. Firstly heat oven to 345F.

2. In a bowl, combine the eggs, coconut milk, vanilla, coconut oil, cocoa and sweetener and stir.

3. In a different bowl, mix the baking soda, shredded coconut and almond flour.

4. Join the content of both bowls together and transfer into a baking dish (square-shaped).

5. Bake for about 40 minutes and allow it to cool for about 20 minutes prior to serving.

6. It should be enough for 15 brownies.

Bacon And Vegetable Salad

Ingredients

- Assorted fresh tomatoes (cut into big pieces), 2 pounds

- Peeled avocado (diced), 4

- Pre-cooked bacon (cut into big pieces), 24 slices

- Washed mixed greens (dried), 6 cups

- Mayonnaise, 1 cup

- Cracked fresh pepper and salt to taste

Preparation

1. Combine all the ingredients inside a bowl; add a little pepper and salt. Serve!

Coconut Cream Chips

Ingredients

- 2big egg whites

- Vanilla, ½ teaspoon

- Tartar cream, 1/8 teaspoon

- Salt, ¼ teaspoon

- Erythritol, ½ cup

- Dried coconut, chopped, 8 ounces (unsweetened)

- Softened cream cheese, 4 cups

- Heavy cream, 1 ounce

- Sugar free White Chocolate Syrup (Da Vinci brand), 1 ounce

- Chocolate Chips (Enjoy Life Semi-Sweet Brand), 1 ounce

Preparation

1. Firstly heat the oven to 320F. Then use parchment paper to line two big cookie sheets. In a very clean, big mixing bowl, mix cream of tartar, vanilla, salt and egg whites, using an electric mixer set to high speed the tips curl (i.e. soft tips form). Gently put the erythritol, at a rate of 1 tablespoon at once, making sure to beat till stiff tips form (i.e. the tips will be erect). Add the coconut.

2. Mix the heavy cream and cream cheese till the batter is smooth. Add the syrup and stir properly. Put the coconut mixture in thirds till it combines. Add chocolate chips.

3. Put the coconut mixture in heaps with the help of a little ice cream scoop (bowl of 1.20-inch size), and place them already prepared cookie sheets. Put in different racks into the oven. Bake for about 17-22 minutes. Put off the oven; allow the cookies to dry inside the oven for about 25 minutes before transferring to a wire rack to cool off.

4. Store in a single-layered sealed container at room temperature for a maximum of 5 days.

Oven-Baked Zucchini flakes

Ingredients

- Olive Oil or coconut oil

- 1 pack Zucchinis

- Paprika, as preferred

- Salt, as preferred

Preparation

1. Preheat the oven to 250 degrees.

2. Chop the zucchinis into fine slices.

3. Pour the zucchinis into a medium-sized mixing bowl and add the oil, paprika and salt. Combine it together properly. Use little olive oil so as not to make it soggy. Also use moderate salt because the zucchini will reduce in size once it is baked.

4. Use parchment paper or aluminum foil to line the inside of the baking sheet.

5. Arrange the zucchinis on the baking sheet in a way that they don't touch each other.

6. Bake for half an hour.

7. Remove the zucchini chips and see if they are done. Toss them over until they are uniformly done.

8. Bake for another half an hour or until it becomes crispy, but check constantly on them so they don't get overcooked.

9. When they turn crispy, remove from oven and allow them to cool down for a few minutes before serving. Eat at once before they become stale after a few hours.

Easy Crock-Pot Beef Chili

Ingredients

- 15 ounces diced tomatoes in juice, canned

- ½ pound ground beef, boiled

- 30 ounces tomato juice, 2 cans

- ¾ Hungarian wax and ½ green peppers

- ½ cup diced green pepper

- 1 tablespoon organic cumin

- 2 medium onions, diced

- 2 rib celery, diced

- 2 tablespoons organic chili powder

- 1 teaspoon powdered Black Pepper

- 2 teaspoons sea salt

- Grated red pepper, if desired

Preparation

1. Mix together all the ingredients in a crock pot and boil on low heat for about 8 or more hours.

2. Top with the sour cream, cheese, avocado, diced raw onion, and so on, as preferred.

3. Serve with my Grain Free Buttermilk Biscuits, Gluten Free Blue Corn Muffins, or Paleo Grain Free Everything Rolls.

Creamy Chicken Salad

Ingredients

Salad ingredients

• Cooked chicken (minced), 3 cups

• Celery (minced), 1 cup

• Green onion (sliced), 1 cup

Dressing ingredients

• Softened cream cheese, 4 ounces

• Mayonnaise, 4ounces

• Dried tarragon, 2 teaspoon

• Dried thyme, 1 teaspoon

• Pepper and salt

Preparation

1. Mix mayonnaise and cream cheese and, stir till it is smooth.

2. Put the seasoning and mix till it is smooth.

Finished Salad:

3. Mix the ingredients for the salad and add dressing to taste, stir to coat the ingredients. Eat from the mixing bowl or wrap in lettuce leaves.

Baked Low-Carb Cross Buns

Ingredients

Hot Cross Buns (Low Carb)

• Coconut flour, 1 cup

• Psyllium husks, 1 cup

• Baking powder, 2 teaspoons

• Granulated stevia (or your preferred sweetener), 3 tablespoons

• Salt, 1 teaspoon

• Mixed spice, 1 teaspoon

• Cinnamon, 1 teaspoon

• Ground cloves, 1 teaspoon

• 6 eggs

• Boiling water, 2 cups (500ml)

• Chocolate chips or cacao nibs or raisins (not compulsory)

Icing

• Erythritol or stevia icing mix

• Water adequate to prepare smooth paste

Preparation

Low Carb Hot Cross Buns

1. Put dry ingredients together in a mixing bowl and mix.

2. Put in the eggs and stir.

3. Pour the boiling water till the mixture has combined equally.

4. Roll into 8 balls of same size then put on a baking tray.

5. Bake in an oven that has fan at 170C/338F for about 25-35 minutes the middle of the buns is cooked and the outside is brown.

Icing

1. Use stevia icing mix to make a cross sign on the hot buns.

Creamy Deviled Eggs

Ingredients

- 8 big eggs

- Mayonnaise, 1/3 cup

- Melted butter, 1 tablespoon

- Yellow mustard, ¼ teaspoon

- White onion, diced, 1/3 cup

- White pepper, 1/3 teaspoon

- Salt, ½ teaspoon

Preparation

1. Pour cold water in a big pot till it is full, and then place the eggs. Allow to boil, and cook for about 8 minutes.

2. Bring the pot down from heat, and allow it to cool for extra 5 minutes.

3. Carefully drain the hot water so as to avoid the eggs falling off.

4. Retain the eggs in the pot and pour cool water to refill the pot. Allow the eggs to cool in the water for about 4-8 minutes.

5. Remove the eggs, dry them and peel.

6. As soon as eggs are peeled, use a thin knife to divide them lengthwise into two.

7. Set a glass bowl aside, extract the cooked yolks and put them in the bowl.

8. Place the white shells on a deviled egg holder or a plate then keep it aside.

9. Crush the yolks with a fork.

10. Add the rest of the ingredients and the mayonnaise to the yolk, and stir properly. Taste and add spice as desired.

11. Use the yolk mixture to fill the cavities of the egg whites with the help of a teaspoon.

12. Cover and store in the refrigerator till it is time to serve.

Paleo Sautéed Orange And Shrimp sauce

Ingredients

- 1½ tablespoon olive oil or ghee

- 1 pounds large shrimp, skinned and deveined

- 2 ¼ tablespoons orange juice, fresh juiced

- ¾ tablespoon arrowroot powder

- 1¼ tablespoon honey

- 1¼ tablespoon coconut aminos

- 1½ tablespoon chili garlic sauce

- ½ tablespoon rice vinegar

- 3 garlic cloves, chopped

- ¾ tablespoon fresh ginger, chopped

Preparation

1. Put the shrimp in a bowl and coat with arrowroot powder. Ensure the shrimp is uniformly coated.

2. Combine the honey, orange juice, rice vinegar coconut aminos, and chili garlic sauce inside a medium bowl.

3. Heat the ghee or olive oil in a big non-stick skillet over medium heat.

4. Stir in the garlic and ginger. Keep stirring for about 10-15 seconds until the garlic becomes scented.

5. Pour in the shrimp and boil for about 3 minutes. Stir in the sauce and boil for another 2 minutes.

6. Take out the shrimp using a slotted spoon.

7. Keep stirring the sauce for additional 2 to 4 minutes until it becomes thick.

8. Sprinkle over the shrimp.

9. Serve on top of fried cauliflower rice or baby spinach.

Baked Italian Crusty Beef

Ingredients

For the Crust:

• Ground beef (with fat removed), 2 pounds

• Mixed dried herbs, 3 tablespoons

• Fresh (or dried) basil, 2 tablespoons

• Garlic, 2cloves (diced)

• Salt, 1 teaspoon

• ½ tsp black pepper

Recommended toppings (1/3 cup of each):

• Tomato sauce

• Paprika, sliced

• Tomatoes (sundried), chopped

• Artichoke hearts (either packed in oil or canned), diced

• Olives, (whichever you prefer), chopped

• Arugula leaves

• Fresh basil (to garnish)

Preparation

1. Firstly heat oven to 392F (200C).

2. Mix all the ingredients to be used for crust in a big bowl- basil, dried herbs, garlic, ground beef, pepper and salt.

3. Share the meat into two parts. Put one half of the meat into a round pie pan of 8". Do same to the second half of the meat.

4. Allow to bake for 18-20 minutes or until properly cooked. Bring down from the oven and drain any liquid found in the pan.

5. Add pepper and tomato sauce, and then bake for 7 minutes. Then, remove the crust and add the remaining toppings - artichokes, arugula leaves, olives and sundried tomatoes. Afterwards, chop into 5 pieces on the cutting board.

Spicy Ground Pork Tacos

Ingredients

• Ground pork (around 20 ounces), 600g

• Powdered garlic, 1 teaspoon

• Onion powder, 1 teaspoon

• Sea salt, 1 teaspoon

• Cumin, ½ teaspoon

• Pepper (ground), ½ teaspoon

• Salsa, 7 tablespoons

• Lettuce leaves, about 7

• Red peppers or onions or avocado or chopped green peppers etc. to top taco with

Preparation

1. Manually mix the ground pork and all the spices (excluding the salsa) in a little bowl.

2. Set oven to average heat and put the meat in a frying pan. Ensure you dismantle any big pieces of meat and stir the meat continually.

3. Drain fat from the frying pan as soon as the meat is tender.

4. Put in the salsa and combine.

5. Use the lettuce wraps to wrap the meat and add your preferred taco toppings.

Cinnamon Ginger Chai

Ingredients

- 1¼ tablespoon grass-fed butter

- 3 cups of hot, organic black tea, strong-brewed

- ½ teaspoon powdered cinnamon

- 1½ tablespoon organic coconut oil

- A few drops of stevia or a teaspoon of honey

- ½ teaspoon powdered ginger

Preparation

Combine together the entire ingredients in a blender and blend on high heat until the mixture is bubbly and emulsified. Drain into two cups and serve while hot.

Vegan Falafel And Tahini Stew

Ingredients

- 3 big eggs

- 1½ cup uncooked cauliflower, squashed

- 1¼ tablespoon powdered cumin

- 1 clove garlic, chopped

- 1 cup powdered slivered almonds

- ¾ tablespoon powdered coriander

- ¾ teaspoon cayenne pepper

- 1 1/3 teaspoon kosher salt

- 4 tablespoon coconut flour

- 3 tablespoon fresh parsley, sliced

Tahini sauce:

- 4 tablespoon water

- 1 teaspoon salt

- 1 ½ tablespoon lemon juice

- 3 tablespoon tahini paste

- 2 cloves garlic, chopped

Preparation

1. To prepare the cauliflower chop it up using a knife, then pour into a food processor or and puree until it's squashed but still retains a grainy quality.

2. Puree the almonds using the food processor also, ensure it is partially grainy to touch.

3. Mix together the powdered cauliflower and almonds in a small mixing bowl. Pour in the remaining ingredients and mix together till well combined.

4. Heat half the olive and half the grape seed oil until warm. While heating the oil, divide the mixture into 8 three-inch patties a little bit thick.

5. Stir-fry them in batches for about 4 minutes per side until well browned on both sides. Transfer to a paper towel-lined plate to drain any surplus oil.

6. Serve with the tahini sauce and garnish with a tomato or parsley if preferred.

7. To prepare the tahini sauce: combine all the ingredients in a mixing bowl. Add a little more water if you prefer it lighter.

Quick Meaty Spaghetti Squash

Ingredients

- Butter, 3 tablespoons

- White onion (diced), 1

- Spaghetti sauce (low sugar), 1½ jar

- Cooked ground beef (or Italian sausage), crushed, 2 cups

- Granulated garlic, 1 teaspoon

- Italian seasoning, 1 teaspoon

- Cooked spaghetti squash, 4 cups

- Pepper and salt

- Parmesan (not compulsory)

Preparation

1. At average-high heat, melt butter in an average-sized saucepan.

2. Put the onion and fry briefly till it is semi-transparent.

3. Add meat and spaghetti sauce, mix, and cook for about 4-5 minutes, decreasing the heat to medium.

4. Put in the Italian seasoning and granulated garlic and stir to combine.

5. Simmer for around 7 minutes, whilst stirring intermittently.

6. Put a cup of the cooked squash and stir to combine.

7. Add squash gradually and mix till the consistence is like that of a creamy casserole.

8. Use Parmesan to garnish. Serve right away.

Coconut Oil Bonbon

Ingredients

• Virgin coconut oil (cold pressed and softened), 2 cups

• Vanilla extract, 2 teaspoons

• Sugar (or preferred sweetener), 3teaspoons

• Celtic sea salt, 1 teaspoon

• Organic cocoa powder (unsweetened), 5 tablespoons

• Almond (or any nut) butter, 3 tablespoons

• Dry coconut (unsweetened), not compulsory

Preparation

1. In a food processor or bowl, combine all the ingredients till it forms a smooth mixture.

2. Use a tablespoon to scoop the mixture onto dry coconut, or parchment paper or waxed.

3. Place in a refrigerator till the candies are hardened, then refrigerate in a sealed container.

Raspberry Fudge pottage

Ingredients

- Softened cream cheese, 2ounces

- Diced Lindt chocolate (90%), 1-2 ounce bar

- Erythritol powder, ½ cup (or as desired)

- Heavy cream 1/3 cup

- Sugar-free raspberry syrup (Monin brand), 1 tablespoon

Preparation

Put the diced chocolate and the cream cheese inside a double boiler (or in a heatproof dish placed on top a pot of boiling water). Stir properly until it is almost fully melted. Put the sweetener and mix till it is smooth and has fully combined. Remove the double boiler and allow it to cool. Wait till the mixture has cooled a little before putting the syrup and heavy cream, and then proceed to stir till the mixture is thick and uniform in consistence. This process requires patience because if cream is added while mixture is still hot it will cause the chocolate to separate.

Stir-fried Chicken Liver with Kale Salad

Ingredients

CHICKEN LIVER

- 2 medium onions or young white onion

- 6 ounces of chicken livers, remove veins and ligaments

- Sea salt and black pepper

- 2½ tablespoons of butter or ghee

KALE SALAD

- 2¼ tablespoons organic apple cider vinegar

- 5 ounces of baby kale leaves

- Sea salt to taste

Preparation

CHICKEN LIVER

1. Dissolve the butter or ghee in a medium-sized skillet.

2. Stir in the onion chopped thinly and sauté slowly on a low heat until tender.

3. Pat the livers dry using a paper towel or cloth.

4. Increase the heat to high then pour in the chicken livers.

5. Stir-fry one side for about 5 minutes before flipping onto the second side.

6. Stir-fry for another 2 or 3 minutes until it is adequately browned but still pink within.

7. Season generously with black pepper and sea salt.

KALE SALAD

8. While cooking the liver, wash the baby kale.

9. Pat the kale dry as well.

10. Use a good kitchen knife to slice it into small bits.

11. Pour the kale into a bowl and mix together with the apple cider vinegar and salt.

12. Serve together at once.

Baked Pumpkin Cookies

Ingredients

- Macadamia nut butter, 12g

- Pumpkin puree (unsweetened, canned), 10g

- Butter, 5g

- Cinnamon (ground), ½ gram

- Baking powder, 0.30g

- Baking soda, 0.30g

- Vanilla extracts (pure), 0.30g

- Egg whites, 8g, whisked into stiff tips

- Liquid stevia, 3 drops (or sweetener of your choice)

Preparation

1. Firstly heat the oven to 360F. Use parchment paper to line a baking sheet.

2. Combine the first 7 ingredients thoroughly to make a smooth batter. Put desired sweetener.

3. Combine the egg whites into the batter. The egg whites may not combine fully but it's no problem.

4. Scoop the batter to lined cookie sheet in spoonfuls and bake for just less than 12 minutes.

Oven-Baked Eggs and Bacon

Ingredients

- Butter, 1 tablespoon

- 2 big eggs

- Cheddar cheese (grated), ½ cup

- Heavy cream, (lukewarm), ½ cup

- Cooked bacon (crushed), 4 slices

- Pepper and salt

Preparation

1. Firstly heat the oven to 345F. Line the inside with 2 little ceramic or glass ramekins of 6 ounce sizes.

2. Into each of the ramekin, break one egg.

3. Use 1/3 cup of heated and 1/3 cup of cheese to coat each egg, then spice up with pepper and salt.

4. Fill a pan with water sufficient to come up to half of the sides of the ramekins, then place ramekins in it.(this is easily achieved by placing the ramekin-filled pan on the oven first, then gradually pouring the water.)

5. Bake till the eggs are fully done and the cheese melted. This would take about 12 minutes.

6. Over each egg, crush a couple slices of cooked bacon, and serve right away.

Paleo Chocolate Keto Gelatin Pudding

Ingredients

- Full fat canned coconut milk, 1 cup

- Organic cocoa or powdered cacao, 1 tablespoon

- Stevia powder extract, ¼ teaspoon

- Maple syrup or honey, 1 tablespoon

- Gelatin (high quality), ½ tablespoon

- Water, 1 tablespoon

Preparation

1. Put the cocoa, sweetener and coconut milk in a pan over average heat and use a whisk to mix.

2. In a small bowl, mix water and gelatin.

3. Dissolve the gelatin in the pan making sure to stir it.

4. As soon as the coconut milk mixture gets warm, put them in two pudding cups or ramekins.

5. Refrigerate for 35-50 minutes or the freezer to set faster.

6. Serve.

Crème Buttery Scallops

Ingredients

- 9 ounces crème fraiche or heavy cream

- 2 ½ tablespoons ghee

- 2 teaspoons garam masala

- 1 cup chopped shallot

- 1 pound sea scallops

- 2 ½ teaspoons fresh ginger paste

- 2 ¼ teaspoons fresh garlic paste

- 1/3 teaspoon salt

- ½ cup tomato paste

- ½ teaspoon powdered cinnamon

- ½ teaspoon powdered cumin

- A dash of cayenne pepper

- Fresh cilantro, optional

Preparation

1. Using a big wok pan or skillet, heat the oil over medium heat. Pour in the shallot and stir-fry, stirring repeatedly until it begins to become tender. Stir in the ginger paste, garam masala, garlic paste, salt, tomato paste, cumin, cayenne and cinnamon, and then boil for an extra 3 to 5 minutes till it becomes thick, and the flavors tasty.

2. Stir in the scallops and crème fraiche, and boil for about 5 minutes or until the scallops are properly done. Top with the fresh cilantro and serve.

Roasted Gouda Alfredo Pottage

Ingredients

- Butter, 2 tablespoons

- Heavy cream, ½ cup

- Egg yolk from 1 big egg

- Smoked gouda cheese (freshly grated), 1 cup

- Paprika, ¼ teaspoon

- Ground nutmeg, ¼ teaspoon

- Pepper and salt to taste

Preparation

1. In an average-sized frying pan, melt the butter at average heat.

2. Put the egg yolk and cream, mix and then cook for an additional for 3-5 minutes, with the heat set to medium low.

3. Mix in the grated cheese. Simmer for around 3 minutes, with repeated stirring.

4. Serve right away or seal then store in the refrigerator.

Buttery Mayonnaise Squash

Ingredients

- Egg yolks (organic), 4

- Lemon juice (freshly squeezed), 4 teaspoons

- Dijon mustard, 2 teaspoons

- Vinegar (white wine), 2 teaspoons

- Sea salt

- Melted butter, ½ cup

- Light olive oil or walnut oil or macadamia, 1 cup

Preparation

1. In the bowl of a food processor, put the lemon juice, salt, vinegar and egg yolk and blend for several seconds to mix.

2. Melt the butter to liquid state, but not excessively hot. Mix in the oil.

3. While the food processor is still running, gradually pour the melted butter/oil mixture into the yolk mixture a little at a time, till the mixture begins to emulsify and stiffen. This would take around 3 minutes.

4. Pour a teaspoon of hot water to the mayonnaise to thin it if it becomes very thick.

5. Taste and add spices as necessary.

Creamy Spinach Sauce

Ingredients

- Raw spinach, 8 ounces

- White onion (diced), ¼ cup

- Shallot (diced), ¼ cup

- Garlic (chopped), 1 clove

- Butter, 1 tablespoon

- Heavy cream, ¼ cup

- Nutmeg, ½ teaspoon

- Pepper and salt to taste

Preparation

1. Put butter in a big skillet.

2. Put the shallots, garlic and diced onion. Fry briefly for around 6-8 minutes or till the onions are tender.

3. Put in the spinach leaves.

4. Briefly fry at average heat with intermittent stirring, making sure to flip the leaves so as to fry both sides of the leaves while frying the whole pile. This mixes the onions also.

5. Secure the lid of the skillet and allow the spinach mixture to boil for around 4 minutes. Stir repeatedly till the spinach is limp and well cooked.

6. Put the nutmeg and cream and combine by stirring. Cook for around 2-3 minutes extra in order thicken the cream.

7. Add pepper and salt as desired.

Browned Cauliflower Tortilla Chips

Ingredients

- 3 medium eggs

- 1 head of cauliflower riced

- Pepper and salt to taste

Preparation

1. Preheat the oven to 375 degrees and use parchment paper to line the inside of the baking tray.

2. Remove the stem of 1 head of cauliflower, slice and pulse until it becomes slightly finer than rice.

3. Put the riced cauliflower in microwave bowl and microwave for about 2 minutes then stir, microwave for another 2 minutes and stir again then put drain out the surplus water using a dish towel.

4. Put the drained cauliflower inside the bowl and pour in the 3 eggs, pepper and salt and then combine until properly blended.

5. Divide the mixture into 6 small reasonably flat circles and spread on a baking sheet.

6. Bake in the oven for about 10 minutes then remove and gently pry them from the parchment paper, flip and place them back in the oven for another 5-7 minutes.

7. When properly done put them on a wire rack and allow it to cool a little.

8. Place a small saucepan on medium heat and pour the tortillas into the saucepan pressing down a bit and allow them to brown as you desire.

9. Serve.

Feta and Bacon Dressing

Ingredients

- Olive oil (organic, cold pressed), 1 cup

- Red wine vinegar, 1 cup

- Garlic, diced, 2 cloves

- Feta cheese (or gorgonzola or blue cheese), crushed, 3 ounces

- Thin bacon, (cooked and crushed), 6 slices

Preparation

1. Mix the garlic, vinegar, feta and oil in a blender and blend till it is properly mixed. Transfer the mixture into a glass bowl. Add the crushed bacon and stir.

2. Serve with vegetable salad, avocado, fruit salad, sliced tomatoes or pork chops.

Stir-fry Beans With Green Bacon

Ingredients

- Handful boiled bacon, sliced into pieces

- 1 small onion, finely chopped

- 1 lb green beans

- Bacon grease or coconut oil

- Salt or GF tamari soy sauce to taste

- 1¼ tablespoon of salt

Preparation

1. Put the green beans inside a pot of boiling water and add a tablespoon of salt. Cook for about 10 minutes or until the green beans become soft enough.

2. Boil the bacon if it's raw.

3. Stir-fry the chopped onion in bacon grease using a frying pan until it becomes translucent. Pour in the drained green beans and boil for about 5 minutes.

4. Stir in the bacon pieces and the salt or tamari sauce to taste.

If you enjoyed reading this book please endeavor to leave a positive review at the customer review section below.

For more of my awesome cookbooks and recipes please visit my author central page:

amazon.com/author/virginiacaldwell

ABOUT THE BOOK

Are you scared of looking in the mirror?

Are you tired of hating the way you look?

Are you prepared to rapidly melt away lumps of fat off your body and maintain a healthy smart look for life?

Trying to be healthy is tough and sometimes frustrating.

But embarking on a ketogenic diet which combines a personalized carbohydrate control, limited protein consumption, and real food-based fats can give you the therapeutic effects needed to burn off chunks of excessive fats from your body.

Consumption of low-carb diets together with high fat diet consumption creates a potent metabolism in the body that is capable of healing a vast range of health conditions and not limited to:

- Lower blood pressure
- Epilepsy
- cardiovascular disease
- Aid weight loss (obesity)
- Metabolic syndrome
- Polycystic ovarian syndrome
- Aid the treatment of Alzheimer's disease
- It is also favorable for individuals suffering with type 2 diabetes who are not on insulin.

This Ketogenic Diet Cookbook Will Teach You How To Make These Enticing Dishes Among Others:

- Baked Sugar Detox Cookies
- Barbecued Lemon-spiced Sardines
- Marinated Oven-Baked Salmon
- Lamb with Rhubarb Stew
- Carne Asada In Crock Pot
- Asian Beef And Broccoli Slaw
- Fat Bomb Easter Egg Cookies
- Vegan Cauliflower And Pizza Crust
- Curried Chicken And Salad

You will find dishes with their step-by-step preparation guide that will aid you in producing more ketones and on your way to feeling amazing.